Keto Honey Alternative Recipes

Table of Contents

TABLE OF CONTENTS 2

DISCLAIMER 4

INTRODUCTION 5

KETO HONEY, DRESSINGS, DIPS ETC. 7

KETO "HONEY" BREAD AND BREAKFAST RECIPES 30

KETO "HONEY" SNACK AND APPETIZER RECIPES 44

KETO "HONEY" LUNCH RECIPES 54

KETO "HONEY" DINNER RECIPES 73

KETO "HONEY" DESSERT RECIPES 101

CONCLUSION 117

Disclaimer

Copyright © 2020

All Rights Reserved.

No part of this book can be transmitted or reproduced in any form including print, electronic, photocopying, scanning, mechanical or recording without prior written permission from the author.

While the author has taken utmost efforts to ensure the accuracy of the written content, all readers are advised to follow information mentioned herein at their own risk. The author cannot be held responsible for any personal or commercial damage caused by information. All readers are encouraged to seek professional advice when needed.

Introduction

Many people wonder if honey is keto or not. Before we get into that let us understand what honey is. The busy little bees make honey, and raw honey has many nutritional benefits. This ingredient is one of the widely known substitutes for sugar and is packed with antioxidants. While both raw honey and sugar have the sugar molecules, fructose and glucose respectively, our bodies digest them differently.

Bees add an enzyme to raw honey, which breaks the sugars down into smaller, easily digestible components. Our body burns these sugar molecules to produce energy. With regular sugar, our body needs to do the work. It needs to produce enzymes to break the molecules apart before it stores the sugars as energy. This gives rise to the question – is honey keto?

What most people worry about is whether eating honey will throw them out of ketosis. You need to remember that your body stays in ketosis if you eat between 25 and 50 grams of carbohydrates every day. If you are active, you can eat more than 100 grams of carbohydrates each day and still stay in ketosis. If you consume honey in moderation, you can stay in ketosis.

As mentioned earlier, raw honey is abundant in different minerals and vitamins, including pantothenic acid, riboflavin, niacin, thiamin, magnesium, copper, calcium, potassium, phosphorus, manganese, zinc, sodium and Vitamin B6. When you replace regular sugar with raw honey, you gain many health benefits, including improved energy, weight loss, increase in antioxidants in your body, antibacterial effects and more.

So, if you love adding some sweet to your dishes, avoid sugar and use raw honey instead. If you are worried about the taste, don't be – raw honey adds both flavor and nutrition to your food unlike sugar. This book has some delicious recipes you can use to incorporate honey to your diet. The instructions are simple, and all the ingredients used can be found in your pantry or the supermarket. If you love sticky, sweet chicken and desserts, use the recipes in the book. You have recipes for every meal of the day.

Thank you for purchasing the book. I hope you enjoy the recipes.

Keto Honey, Dressings, Dips etc.

Keto Honey (Sugar-free Honey Syrup) #1

Preparation time: 5 minutes

Cooking time: 1 – 2 minutes

Number of servings: 24 (1 ½ cups)

Nutritional values per serving: 1 tablespoon

Calories – 32

Fat – 0.2 g

Total Carbohydrate – 13.7 g

Net Carbohydrate – 1.6 g

Fiber – 12.1 g

Protein – 0.5 g

Ingredients:

- 4 tablespoons bee pollen
- 1 cup Sukrin Fiber Syrup Clear

- 3 – 4 tablespoons water

Directions:

1. Add water into a saucepan. Place the saucepan over low flame. When the water is warm, turn off the heat.
2. Add bee pollen in the smaller blender jar. Pour 1 ½ - 2 tablespoons of warm water over the bee pollen. Wait for about 10 minutes.
3. Give short pulses and blend until smooth.
4. Add more water if the mixture is too thick. Pour sukrin syrup and blend until smooth.
5. Pour into a jar. Fasten the lid and store at room temperature. If you want to store it for longer period of time, place the jar in the refrigerator. It can last for 3 – 4 months.
6. Use this "honey" instead of regular honey in your Ketogenic diet. You can experiment by replacing this "honey" in many recipes like smoothies, desserts, beverages etc.

Keto Honey (Sugar-free Honey Syrup) #2

Preparation time: 2 minutes

Cooking time: 10 – 12 minutes

Number of servings: 32

Nutritional values per serving: 1 tablespoon

Calories – 1

Fat – 0 g

Total Carbohydrate – 0 g

Net Carbohydrate – 0 g

Fiber – 0 g

Protein – 0 g

Ingredients:

- 2 cups cold, filtered water
- 12 tablespoons xylitol or erythritol
- 2 teaspoons honey flavoring (optional)
- ¼ teaspoon xanthan gum or glucomannan
- ¼ teaspoon mineral salt

- 10 drops yellow food coloring (optional)

Directions:

1. Add ½ cup cold water and xanthan gum into a bowl and whisk well.
2. Add 1 ½ cups cold water, xylitol and mineral salt into a saucepan. Place the saucepan over medium flame. Let the mixture come to a boil.
3. Stir often until the sweetener dissolves completely.
4. Add the xanthan gum mixture, stirring constantly. When the mixture is thick, turn off the heat. Do not make it too thick, as it will cool, it will become thicker.
5. Add honey flavoring and food coloring. Whisk well. Transfer into an airtight container and refrigerate until use.

Keto Honey Vinaigrette

Preparation time: 2 minutes

Cooking time: 0 minutes

Number of servings: 12 (1 tablespoon each)

Nutritional values per serving: 1 tablespoon

Calories – 83.25

Fat – 9 g

Total Carbohydrate – 0.77 g

Net Carbohydrate – 0.77 g

Fiber – 0 g

Protein – 0.01 g

Ingredients:

- ½ cup olive oil
- ½ tablespoon keto honey syrup
- ¼ cup apple cider vinegar
- ¼ teaspoon stevia

Directions:

1. Add oil, keto honey syrup, apple cider vinegar and stevia into the beaker of the immersion blender.
2. Blend until well combined.
3. Pour into a jar. Fasten the lid and store at room temperature. If you want to store it for longer period of time, place the jar in the refrigerator. It can last for a week.
4. Shake the jar well before using.

Keto Honey Mustard Dressing

Preparation time: 5 minutes

Cooking time: 0 minutes

Number of servings: 16 (2 cups)

Nutritional values per serving: 2 tablespoons

Calories – 38

Fat – 2.5 g

Total Carbohydrate – 0.5 g

Fiber – 0 g

Protein – 0.4 g

Ingredients:

- 1 cup full-fat sour cream
- ½ cup Dijon mustard
- 2 tablespoons granular erythritol
- ½ cup water
- 2 tablespoons apple cider vinegar

Directions:

1. Add sour cream, granular erythritol, water, apple cider vinegar and Dijon mustard into an airtight container. Stir until well combined.
2. Close the lid of the container and refrigerate until use. It can last for 2 weeks.

"Honey" Mustard Sauce

Preparation time: 5 minutes

Cooking time: 0 minutes

Number of servings: 8

Nutritional values per serving: 1/8 recipe

Calories – 108

Fat – 10 g

Total Carbohydrate – 3.3 g

Net Carbohydrate – 0.3 g

Fiber – 3 g

Protein – 0.8 g

Ingredients:

- ½ cup keto friendly full-fat mayonnaise
- 8 teaspoons keto honey
- 8 teaspoons Dijon mustard

Directions:

1. Combine mayonnaise, keto honey and Dijon mustard in an airtight container.
2. Close the lid of the container and refrigerate until use. It can last for 2 weeks.

Keto BBQ Sauce

Preparation time: 15 minutes

Cooking time: 45 minutes

Number of servings: 40 – 50 servings (5 – 6 cups)

Nutritional values per serving: 2 tablespoons

Calories – 28

Fat – 2.3 g

Total Carbohydrate – 1.6 g

Net Carbohydrate – 1 g

Fiber – 0.6 g

Protein – 0.33 g

Ingredients:

- 2 cans (6 ounces each) tomato paste
- 1 can apple cider vinegar
- 2/3 cup Sukrin gold brown sugar substitute or monk fruit sweetener
- 2 teaspoons minced garlic

- 1 teaspoon dried thyme
- 2 teaspoons Hickory liquid smoke
- ½ teaspoon salt
- 8 tablespoons butter
- ¼ teaspoon ground cloves
- 1 ½ tablespoons ground chipotle pepper
- 4 teaspoons Worcestershire sauce
- 1 teaspoon freshly ground pepper
- 4 cans water (use the empty can of tomato paste to measure)
- 1 can red wine vinegar (use the empty can of tomato paste to measure)
- 1 cup diced onion

Directions:

1. Add tomato paste, water, apple cider vinegar, sugar substitute, onion, garlic, cloves, thyme and chipotle pepper into a saucepan.
2. Place the saucepan over medium flame. Stir frequently until well combined and smooth.

3. When the mixture begins to boil, lower the heat and cook for about 45 minutes or until the thickness you desire is achieved, stirring occasionally. Turn off the ingredients.
4. Add Worcestershire sauce, pepper, liquid smoke, butter and salt. Blend with an immersion blender until you get a smooth sauce.
5. Let it rest for 8 – 9 hours. Taste the sauce. If you are happy with the taste, transfer into an airtight container else add seasonings and mix well before adding into the container.
6. Refrigerate until use. It can last for 10 days.

Keto Chick- Fil-A Sauce

Preparation time: 5 minutes

Cooking time: 0 minutes

Number of servings: 8

Nutritional values per serving: 3 tablespoons

Calories – 127

Fat – 10.5 g

Total Carbohydrate – 3.5 g

Net Carbohydrate – 3 g

Fiber – 0.5 g

Protein – 0.5 g

Ingredients:

- ½ cup keto friendly mayonnaise
- 4 tablespoons sugar-free BBQ sauce
- 4 tablespoons sugar-free honey syrup (keto honey)
- 3 tablespoons yellow mustard

- 4 tablespoons lemon juice
- Paprika to taste

Directions:

1. Add mayonnaise, BBQ sauce, keto honey, mustard, lemon juice and paprika into a jar and stir well.
2. Fasten the lid and refrigerate for at least a couple of hours before use. It can last for a week.

Keto "Honey" Mustard

Preparation time: 3 minutes

Cooking time: 0 minutes

Number of servings: 16

Nutritional values per serving:

Calories – 116

Fat – 10.8 g

Total Carbohydrate – 6.1 g

Net Carbohydrate – 0.8 g

Fiber – 0.3 g

Protein – 0.6 g

Ingredients:

- 1 cup keto friendly full-fat mayonnaise
- ½ cup keto honey
- ¼ teaspoon cayenne pepper
- ¼ teaspoon salt
- 2/3 cup yellow mustard

Directions:

1. Combine mayonnaise, keto honey, cayenne pepper, salt and yellow mustard in an airtight container.
2. Close the lid of the container and refrigerate until use. It can last for 2 weeks.

Keto "Honey" Mustard Dressing / Dipping Sauce

Preparation time: 10 minutes

Cooking time: 0 minutes

Number of servings: 10 (2 ½ cups)

Nutritional values per serving: ¼ cup

Calories – 248

Fat – 26.4 g

Total Carbohydrate – 0.11 g

Net Carbohydrate – 0.11 g

Fiber – 0 g

Protein – 1 g

Ingredients:

- 1 ½ cups keto friendly mayonnaise
- ½ cup heavy cream
- 2 tablespoons lemon juice
- ½ teaspoon onion powder

- ¼ teaspoon cayenne pepper
- 1 cup Dijon mustard
- 6 tablespoons swerve confectioners' or lakanto confectioners'
- Pepper to taste
- ½ teaspoon granulated garlic powder
- ½ teaspoon dried tarragon, crushed
- Salt to taste

Directions:

1. Combine mayonnaise, onion powder, cayenne pepper, swerve, pepper, garlic powder, tarragon, salt and Dijon mustard in an airtight container.
2. Add cream, about a tablespoon at a time and whisk well each time.
3. Add vinegar and whisk well.
4. Close the lid of the container and refrigerate for at least 8 – 9 hours before use. It can last for 10 days.

Keto "Honey" Mustard Salad Dressing

Preparation time: 3 minutes

Number of servings: 16

Nutritional values per serving:

Calories – 116

Fat – 10.8 g

Total Carbohydrate – 6.1 g

Net Carbohydrate – 0.8 g

Fiber – 0.3 g

Protein – 0.6 g

Ingredients:

- 1 cup keto friendly full-fat mayonnaise
- ½ cup keto honey
- 2 tablespoons white vinegar
- ¼ teaspoon cayenne pepper
- ¼ teaspoon salt
- 2/3 cup yellow mustard

Directions:

1. Combine mayonnaise, keto honey, vinegar, cayenne pepper, salt and yellow mustard in an airtight container.
2. Close the lid of the container and refrigerate until use. It can last for 2 weeks.

Honey Cinnamon Butter

Preparation time: 10 minutes

Cooking time: 0 minutes

Number of servings: 8

Nutritional values per serving: 1 tablespoon

Calories – 101

Fat – 11 g

Total Carbohydrate – 0 g

Net Carbohydrate – 0 g

Fiber – 0 g

Protein – 0 g

Ingredients:

- ½ cup salted butter, at room temperature
- 25 – 30 drops liquid stevia
- 1 teaspoon powdered cinnamon

Directions:

1. Add butter, cinnamon and stevia into an airtight container and stir until well combined.
2. Close the lid of the container and refrigerate until use. It can last for 1 week.

Keto "Honey" Bread and Breakfast Recipes

"Honey" Almond Biscuits

Preparation time: 15 minutes

Cooking time: 15 – 20 minutes

Number of servings: 30

Nutritional values per serving: 1 biscuit

Calories – 95

Fat – 7 g

Total Carbohydrate – 1 g

Net Carbohydrate – 1 g

Fiber – 0 g

Protein – 5 g

Ingredients:

- 1 cup almond meal or almond flour
- 4 tablespoons butter, melted
- 6 tablespoons keto honey

- 12 ounces finely shredded parmesan cheese
- 4 large eggs, beaten

Directions:

1. Combine almond meal and parmesan cheese in a mixing bowl.
2. Add butter, keto honey and eggs and stir until well combined.
3. Prepare a large baking sheet by lining it with parchment paper. Use 2 baking sheets if required.
4. Scoop the batter into 30 equal portions and drop onto the prepared baking sheet. Leave gap between the biscuits. You should have 30 biscuits in all.
5. Place the baking sheet in an oven that has been preheated to 325°F and bake until golden brown on top. It should take around 15 – 20 minutes.

Keto Honey Wheat Style Bread

Preparation time: 20 minutes

Cooking time: 30 – 35 minutes

Number of servings: 7

Nutritional values per serving: 1 slice

Calories – 84

Fat – 6.4 g

Total Carbohydrate – 3.5 g

Net Carbohydrate – 1 g

Fiber – 2.5 g

Protein – 3.1 g

Ingredients:

- 3 tablespoons ground flaxseeds
- ¼ cup almond flour
- 2 tablespoons whole psyllium husks
- ¼ teaspoon Himalayan pink salt
- ¼ tablespoon swerve granular

- ¼ teaspoon ground cinnamon
- 1 ¼ teaspoons aluminum free baking powder
- 1/8 teaspoon baking soda
- 1/8 cup water
- 2 large eggs
- 1 tablespoon sesame seeds or Everything bagel seasoning (optional)
- 1 tablespoon olive oil
- ¾ tablespoon apple cider vinegar
- 1 ¼ tablespoons hemp hearts

Directions:

1. You need to prepare the oven and loaf pan: Place rack in the center of the oven. Also make sure that the oven is preheated to 350°F.
2. Take a small loaf pan and line it with parchment paper.
3. To mix dry ingredients: Combine ground flaxseeds, almond flour, psyllium husks, salt, swerve, cinnamon, hemp hearts, baking powder and baking soda into a mixing bowl.
4. To mix wet ingredients: Combine apple cider vinegar, olive oil, water and eggs in a bowl. Whisk well.

5. Pour the mixture of wet ingredients into the bowl of dry ingredients and whisk until smooth and free from lumps.
6. Spoon the batter into the loaf pan. Scatter sesame seeds on top.
7. Place the baking dish in the oven and bake until brown on top. It should take around 30 – 35 minutes. Let the bread remain in the baking dish for 10 – 15 minutes.
8. Take out the bread from the loaf pan along with the parchment paper and place on a cooling rack.
9. Once cooled, cut into 7 equal slices and serve.

Keto Honey Cornbread

Preparation time: 5 minutes

Cooking time: 35 minutes

Number of servings: 8

Nutritional values per serving:

Calories – 300

Fat – 27 g

Total Carbohydrate – 8 g

Net Carbohydrate – 4 g

Fiber – 4 g

Protein – 10 g

Ingredients:

- 2 ½ cups blanched almond flour
- 3 tablespoon monk fruit allulose blend
- ½ tablespoon baking powder
- ½ teaspoon sea salt
- 1/3 cup butter, melted + extra to grease

- 3 large eggs
- 1/3 cup unsweetened almond milk
- ½ tablespoon sweet corn extract

Directions:

1. You need to prepare the oven and skillet: Place rack in the center of the oven. Also make sure that the oven is preheated to 350°F.
2. Take a small cast-iron skillet and brush some butter inside the pan.
3. To mix dry ingredients: Combine almond flour, sweetener, baking powder and salt in a mixing bowl.
4. Add butter, eggs and almond milk and whisk until smooth. Add sweet corn extract and stir until well combined.
5. Pour the batter into the prepared skillet. Spread it evenly with a spatula.
6. Place the skillet in the oven and bake until brown on top. It should take around 30 – 35 minutes. Let the bread remain in the skillet for 25 – 30 minutes or until golden brown on top. When you insert a toothpick in the middle of the bread and remove it, it should come out without any particles stuck on it.
7. Cool completely. Cut into 8 equal slices and serve.

Keto Chocolate and "Honey" Granola

Preparation time: 10 minutes

Cooking time: 30 minutes

Number of servings: 8

Nutritional values per serving: ¼ cup

Calories – 135

Fat – 12 g

Total Carbohydrate – 5 g; Net Carbohydrate – 2 g

Fiber – 3 g

Protein – 3 g

Ingredients:

- 2.6 ounces slivered almonds
- ¼ cup keto honey
- 2 tablespoons ghee
- 1.8 ounces coconut flakes
- 2 tablespoons cacao powder
- 1/8 teaspoon salt

Directions:

1. You need to prepare the oven and baking sheet: Place rack in the center of the oven. Also make sure that the oven is preheated to 320°F.
2. Take a small baking sheet and line it with parchment paper. Scatter almonds and coconut flakes on the baking sheet and place it in the oven.
3. Bake for 8 minutes. Stir once after about 4 minutes of baking. Transfer the almonds and coconut flakes into a bowl.
4. Add keto honey, cacao, ghee and salt into a small saucepan. Place the saucepan over medium flame. Stir until smooth. Pour the keto honey mixture into the bowl of almonds. Mix until well coated.
5. Transfer the almond mixture onto the baking sheet. Spread it evenly.
6. Place the baking sheet in the oven and bake for another 15 to 20 minutes. Stir the nut mixture in intervals 5 of minutes, making sure to spread it in a single layer each time you stir.
7. Cool completely. Transfer into an airtight container and store at room temperature.

Keto "Honey" Bunches of Oats Cereal

Preparation time: 5 minutes

Cooking time: 20 minutes

Number of servings: 10

Nutritional values per serving: ½ cup

Calories – 293

Fat – 31 g

Total Carbohydrate – 12 g

Net Carbohydrate – 5 g

Fiber – 7 g

Protein – 9 g

Ingredients:

- 2 cups sliced almonds
- ½ cup chopped pecans
- 4 tablespoons swerve
- 2 tablespoons butter, melted

- 2 cups flaked coconut
- ½ cup flaxseed meal
- ½ cup keto honey or sugar-free pancake syrup
- ½ teaspoon salt

Directions:

1. You need to prepare the oven and baking sheet: Place rack in the center of the oven. Also make sure that the oven is preheated to 350°F.
2. Take a small baking sheet and line it with parchment paper. Add nuts, coconut flakes, sweetener, salt and flaxseed meal into a bowl and toss well.
3. Add keto honey and melted butter and stir until well coated.
4. Transfer the almond mixture onto the baking sheet. Spread it evenly.
5. Place the baking sheet in the oven and bake for 15 to 20 minutes. Stir the nut mixture in intervals of 5 minutes, making sure to spread it in a single layer each time you stir.
6. Cool completely. Break the baked cereal into big chunks. Transfer into an airtight container and store at room temperature.

Keto Almond Flour Pancakes

Preparation time: 10 minutes

Cooking time: 10 minutes

Number of servings: 3

Nutritional values per serving: 1 pancake, without keto honey and other serving options

Calories – 299

Fat – 19.9 g

Total Carbohydrate – 5.6 g

Net Carbohydrate – 2.6 g

Fiber – 3 g

Protein – 7.2 g

Ingredients:

For the wet ingredients:

- 1 egg, at room temperature
- 2 tablespoons coconut oil, melted or use any other oil of your choice, at room temperature

- 3 tablespoons unsweetened vanilla almond milk (or use plain almond milk with 2 to 3 drops of vanilla extract), at room temperature

For dry ingredients:

- ¼ teaspoon baking soda
- ½ cup + 1/8 cup almond flour

To serve:

- Keto honey, as required
- Peanut butter
- Plain, unsalted butter
- Berries of your choice (optional)
- Whipped cream, stevia sweetened (optional)

Directions:

1. To mix dry ingredients: Add almond flour and baking soda into a mixing bowl

and stir until well combined.

2. To mix wet ingredients: Add vanilla almond milk and egg into another bowl and

whisk until well combined.

3. Pour the mixture of wet ingredients into the bowl of dry ingredients and stir until

well combined. The batter should be smooth.

4. Place a nonstick pan over medium-high flame. Spray the pan with cooking spray.

5. Pour ¼ cup of batter on the pan (it would be approximately 1/3 of the batter). In

a minute or so, bubbles will be visible on the pancakes.

6. Cook until the underside is browned, as per your desire. Turn the pancake over

and cook the other side as well.

7. Remove the pancake onto a plate.

8. Repeat steps 5 – 8 and make the remaining pancakes.

9. Spread some butter on top. Drizzle keto honey over the pancakes and serve with

peanut butter or berries or any other keto friendly toppings.

Keto "Honey" Snack and Appetizer Recipes

"Honey" Roasted Peanuts

Preparation time: 10 minutes

Cooking time: 14 minutes

Number of servings: 8 – 9

Nutritional values per serving: ¼ cup

Calories – 259

Fat – 24 g

Total Carbohydrate – 6 g

Net Carbohydrate – 3 g

Fiber – 3 g

Protein – 9 g

Ingredients:

- 2 cups salted, roasted peanuts
- ¼ cup swerve brown
- ¼ cup granulated swerve

- ½ teaspoon vanilla extract
- ¼ cup butter, melted
- ½ teaspoon ground cinnamon

Directions:

1. You need to prepare the oven and baking sheet: Place rack in the center of the oven. Also make sure that the oven is preheated to 325°F.
2. Take a baking sheet and line it with parchment paper.
3. Combine melted butter, swerve brown sugar, vanilla and cinnamon in a bowl.
4. Stir in the peanuts. Once peanuts are well coated with the mixture, spread them on the baking sheet. Scatter granulated swerve over the peanuts.
5. Place the baking sheet in the oven and bake for 10 to 12 minutes. Stir the peanuts in intervals of 5 minutes, making sure to spread it in a single layer each time you stir.
6. Cool completely. Break the baked peanuts into small pieces. Transfer into an airtight container and store at room temperature.

"Honey" Garlic Pork Riblets

Preparation time: 10 minutes

Cooking time: 50 – 60 minutes

Number of servings: 4

Nutritional values per serving: ¼ recipe

Calories – 227

Fat – 16 g

Total Carbohydrate – 1 g

Net Carbohydrate – 0 g

Fiber – 0 g

Protein – 19 g

Ingredients:

- 1 pound pork riblets
- ½ teaspoon minced garlic
- ½ teaspoon minced ginger
- 1 tablespoon white vinegar
- Salt to taste

- ½ can diet cola (splenda or stevia sweetened)
- ½ tablespoon soy sauce
- ½ tablespoon dried onion flakes
- Pepper to taste

Directions:

1. Add pork, garlic, ginger, vinegar, cola, soy sauce, onion flakes and pepper into a saucepan.
2. Place the saucepan over medium flame. When the mixture begins to boil, lower the heat and cook covered, until pork is cooked through.
3. Uncover and cook until you get thick sauce. Remove only the pork from the saucepan (not the sauce). Remove extra fat from the pork.
4. Add salt into the sauce and mix well. Transfer the sauce into a small serving bowl.
5. Place riblets on a serving platter along with sauce.

BBQ Lamb Riblets

Preparation time: 5 minutes

Cooking time: 40 minutes

Number of servings: 3

Nutritional values per serving: 1/3 recipe without coleslaw

Calories – 432

Fat – 24 g

Total Carbohydrate – 4 g

Net Carbohydrate – 3 g

Fiber – 1 g

Protein – 25 g

Ingredients:

- 1 pound lamb riblets, cut into individual ribs
- ¼ teaspoon salt
- ½ ounce keto BBQ sauce
- 1 tablespoon lemon juice
- 1 tablespoon chermoula spice mix

- ½ ounce sugar-free tomato ketchup
- ½ ounce sukrin gold fiber syrup
- ½ tablespoon olive oil

Directions:

1. Sprinkle salt and chermoula spice mix over the riblets and rub it into it. Cover and set aside for 4 – 8 hours.
2. You need to prepare the oven and baking sheet: Place rack in the center of the oven. Also make sure that the oven is preheated to 390°F.
3. Take a baking sheet and line it with parchment paper.
4. Add ketchup, sukrin fiber syrup, BBQ sauce, oil and lemon juice into a bowl and whisk until well combined. Brush a little of this mixture over the riblets and place them on the baking sheet.
5. Place the baking sheet in the oven and bake for 30 to 40 minutes. Brush the sauce mixture over the riblets in intervals of 10 minutes until the meat is cooked and falls off the bone.
6. Serve with keto coleslaw.

Sesame Brittle Bars

Preparation time: 5 minutes

Cooking time: 5 minutes

Number of servings: 3

Nutritional values per serving: 5 bars

Calories – 141

Fat – 11 g

Total Carbohydrate – 3 g

Net Carbohydrate – 0 g

Fiber – 3 g

Protein – 5 g

Ingredients:

- ½ cup sesame seeds
- 1 ½ tablespoon brown sugar substitute
- 1 ½ tablespoons keto honey
- ½ teaspoon vanilla extract (optional)

Directions:

1. You need to prepare the baking sheet: Take a baking sheet and line it with parchment paper.
2. Add keto honey and brown sugar substitute into a pan. Place the pan over medium flame. Stir until well combined. Cook until thick like honey.
3. Stir in vanilla extract.
4. Add sesame seeds and stir well. Turn off the heat.
5. Spread the mixture onto the prepared baking sheet. Spread it as thin as possible.
6. Mark into 15 equal bars, with a knife (dip the knife in water before marking). Let it cool completely.
7. Take a scissors and cut the bars along with parchment paper.
8. Transfer into an airtight container.
9. Peel off the parchment paper just before serving.

Candied Nuts

Preparation time: 5 minutes

Cooking time: 5 minutes

Number of servings: 8

Nutritional values per serving: 1/8 recipe

Calories – 135

Fat – 15 g

Total Carbohydrate – 3 g

Net Carbohydrate – 1 g

Fiber – 2 g

Protein – 2 g

Ingredients:

- 1 ½ cups whole, raw nuts of your choice like almonds, cashews etc.
- ½ tablespoon ground cinnamon
- ½ cup granulated sweetener of your choice like swerve, erythritol etc.

- ½ teaspoon sea salt
- ½ teaspoon honey flavoring
- 2 tablespoons water

Directions:

1. Place a large pan over medium flame. Add swerve, cinnamon, salt and water and mix well. Let it cook for a few minutes, until sweetener dissolves completely. Stir occasionally.
2. Add nuts and stir until the nuts are well coated with the syrup. Turn off the heat and add honey flavoring. Mix well.
3. Transfer onto a plate and let it cool completely.
4. Store in an airtight container until use.

Keto "Honey" Lunch Recipes

Cobb Salad with "Honey" Mustard Vinaigrette

Preparation time: 5 minutes

Cooking time: 15 minutes

Number of servings: 2

Nutritional values per serving: ½ the recipe

Calories – 550

Fat – 39 g

Total Carbohydrate – 10 g

Net Carbohydrate – 4 g

Fiber – 6 g

Protein – 45 g

Ingredients:

For salad:

- 6 ounces bacon

- ½ package (from a 5 ounce package) spinach and arugula blend
- 2 hardboiled eggs, peeled, cut into quarters
- 2 chicken breasts
- 2 ounces cherry tomatoes
- 1 medium avocado, peeled, pitted sliced

For honey mustard vinaigrette:

- ½ tablespoon Dijon mustard
- 1 tablespoon extra-virgin olive oil
- 1/8 teaspoon salt
- ½ tablespoons apple cider vinegar
- 1 teaspoon swerve or erythritol or more to taste

Directions:

1. To make dressing: Add Dijon mustard, oil, salt, apple cider vinegar and swerve into a small jar and close the lid.
2. Shake the jar vigorously for about a minute or until well combined.
3. To cook bacon: Place a pan over medium flame. Add bacon and cook until crisp.

4. Remove bacon with a slotted spoon and place on a plate lined with paper towels. When cool enough to handle, cut into pieces.
5. Add chicken into the same pan and cook until the underside is golden brown. Turn the chicken over and cook the other side until golden brown in color and cooked through inside.
6. Remove chicken from the pan and place on your cutting board. When cool enough to handle, chop the chicken into bite size pieces.
7. To make salad: Add chicken, lettuce, eggs, cherry tomatoes and avocado into a bowl and toss well.
8. Shake the jar of dressing and pour dressing over the salad. Toss well and serve.

Keto "Honey" Mustard Rotisserie Chicken Salad

Preparation time: 5 minutes

Cooking time: 0 minutes

Number of servings: 2

Nutritional values per serving: ½ the recipe

Calories – 324

Fat – 23 g

Total Carbohydrate – 7 g

Net Carbohydrate – 5 g

Fiber – 3 g

Protein – 20 g

Ingredients:

For the salad:

- 1 cup diced rotisserie chicken
- ½ cup halved cherry tomatoes
- 2 cups shredded romaine lettuce

For the dressing:

- 4 teaspoons Dijon mustard
- 2 teaspoons cider vinegar
- Black pepper to taste
- 2 teaspoons sugar-free keto honey
- 2 tablespoons olive oil
- Salt to taste

Directions:

1. To make dressing: Add Dijon mustard, oil, salt, pepper, cider vinegar and keto honey into a small jar and close the lid.
2. Shake the jar vigorously for about a minute or until well combined.
3. To make salad: Add chicken, tomatoes and lettuce into a bowl and toss well. Pour dressing on top. Toss well and serve.

Broccoli "Honey" Salad

Preparation time: 15 minutes

Cooking time: 30 minutes

Number of servings: 4

Nutritional values per serving: 1 cup

Calories – 346

Fat – 23 g

Total Carbohydrate – 5 g

Net Carbohydrate – 3 g

Fiber – 2 g

Protein – 7 g

Ingredients:

For salad:

- 2 ½ cups broccoli florets
- 2 tablespoons diced jalapeño peppers
- 4 slices bacon
- 2 ounces cheddar cheese, shredded

- 1 small red bell pepper, diced
- 1 ½ scallions, diced
- ¾ ounce macadamia nuts, to garnish

For dressing:

- ½ cup mayonnaise
- 1 tablespoon apple cider vinegar
- Pepper to taste
- 1 ½ teaspoons powdered monk fruit sweetener
- Salt to taste

Directions:

1. To make dressing: Add mayonnaise, monk fruit sweetener, salt, pepper and apple cider vinegar into a bowl and stir until well combined. Cover and set aside until the bacon is cooked.
2. To cook bacon: Place a pan over medium flame. Add bacon and cook until crisp.
3. Remove bacon with a slotted spoon and place on a plate lined with paper towels. When cool enough to handle, cut into pieces.

4. To make salad: Add broccoli, jalapeño pepper, scallions, red bell pepper, bacon and cheese into a bowl and toss well.
5. Pour dressing over the salad and fold gently. Chill until you serve.

"Honey" Walnut Shrimp

Preparation time: 10 minutes

Cooking time: 10 minutes

Number of servings: 2

Nutritional values per serving:

Calories – 480

Fat – 40 g

Total Carbohydrate – 21 g

Net Carbohydrate – 1 g

Fiber – 2 g

Protein – 26 g

Ingredients:

For candied walnuts:

- ¼ cup walnuts
- 2 ½ tablespoons brown swerve
- A pinch salt
- ¾ teaspoon water

For shrimp:

- ½ pound large shrimp, peeled, deveined
- Pepper to taste
- ¼ cup coconut oil
- Salt to taste

For sauce:

- 3 tablespoons mayonnaise
- ½ tablespoon heavy cream
- ½ - 1 tablespoon swerve confectioners'
- ½ teaspoon lemon juice

Optional garnishing:

- 1 tablespoon thinly sliced green onion
- Shredded cabbage

Directions:

1. To make candied walnuts: Place a small saucepan over medium flame. Add swerve, salt and water and mix well. Let it cook for a few minutes, until sweetener dissolves completely. Stir occasionally. Let the mixture come to a rolling boil.

2. Add walnuts and stir until the walnuts are well coated with the syrup. Turn off the heat.
3. Transfer onto a plate and let it cool completely.
4. Store in an airtight container until use.
5. To make shrimp: Place a pan over medium flame. Add oil. Once oil melts, place shrimp in the pan and cook until pink on each side.
6. Remove shrimp and place on layers of paper towels, placed over a plate.
7. To make sauce: Add mayonnaise, heavy cream, swerve and lemon juice into a bowl and mix until well incorporated.
8. Add shrimp and toss well. Scatter candied walnuts on top.
9. Garnish with cabbage and green onion and serve.

Keto Honey Mustard Chicken

Preparation time: 5 minutes + marinating time

Cooking time: 30 minutes

Number of servings: 2

Nutritional values per serving:

Calories – 242

Fat – 9.5 g

Total Carbohydrate – 1 g

Net Carbohydrate – 1 g

Fiber – 0 g

Protein – 34 g

Ingredients:

- 2 boneless, skinless chicken breasts
- 1 tablespoon olive oil
- ½ cup keto honey mustard dressing

Directions:

1. Add ¼ cup keto honey mustard dressing into a bowl. Add chicken and stir until chicken is well coated in the dressing.
2. Cover and chill for 1 – 24 hours.
3. Place an ovenproof skillet over medium-high flame. Add oil and let it heat.
4. When the oil is heated, place chicken in the pan and cook until brown on the underside. Turn the chicken over and cook the other side until brown.
5. Turn off the heat and shift the skillet into an oven that has been preheated to 350°F. Once the chicken is well cooked inside, switch off the oven. It should take about 20 minutes.

Keto "Honey" Sriracha Chicken Wings

Preparation time: 10 minutes

Cooking time: 50 minutes

Number of servings: 3

Nutritional values per serving:

Calories – 312

Fat – 20 g

Total Carbohydrate – 12 g

Net Carbohydrate – 3 g

Fiber – 9 g

Protein – 22 g

Ingredients:

<u>For chicken:</u>

- 1.5 pounds chicken wings, cut into drum and flat parts
- ½ teaspoon sea salt
- ½ teaspoon smoked paprika
- 1 tablespoon baking powder

- ½ teaspoon black pepper

For keto "honey" sriracha sauce:

- 2 tablespoons sugar-free caramel syrup like Honest syrup
- ½ tablespoon unseasoned rice vinegar or lime juice
- 1 tablespoon sliced green onion, to serve (optional)
- 1 ½ tablespoon sriracha sauce
- ¼ teaspoon sesame oil
- ½ tablespoon sesame seeds, to serve (optional)

Directions:

1. You need to prepare the oven and baking sheet: Place rack in the center of the oven. Also make sure that the oven is preheated to 425°F.
2. Take a baking sheet and line it with parchment paper.
3. To prepare the chicken: Pat the chicken wings with paper towels until they are dry.
4. Add salt, paprika, baking powder and black pepper into a bowl and mix well. Sprinkle this mixture all over the chicken.
5. Spread the chicken wings on the prepared baking sheet.

6. Place the baking sheet in the oven and bake for 50 to 60 minutes until crisp or as per your preference. Turn the wings over after about 30 minutes of baking.
7. While the wings are baking, make the sauce by combining sugar-free caramel syrup, rice vinegar, sesame oil and sriracha sauce.
8. To serve: Add wings into the sauce and stir to coat.
9. Garnish with sesame seeds and green onion and serve.

Honey Sesame Chicken

Preparation time: 15 minutes

Cooking time: 15 minutes

Number of servings: 6

Nutritional values per serving: 1/6 recipe without serving options

Calories – 297

Fat – 16 g

Total Carbohydrate – 7 g

Net Carbohydrate – 5 g

Fiber – 2 g

Protein – 34 g

Ingredients:

For the chicken:

- 2 pounds chicken thighs, chopped into bite size chunks
- 2 tablespoons arrowroot powder
- Salt to taste
- 2 large eggs

- Black pepper to taste
- 2 tablespoons toasted sesame oil
- 2 tablespoons chopped scallions, to garnish

For the sauce:

- 4 tablespoons coconut aminos
- 4 tablespoons sukrin gold
- 2 teaspoons freshly grated ginger
- 4 tablespoons sesame seeds
- 2 tablespoons toasted sesame oil
- 2 tablespoons white vinegar
- 2 cloves garlic, peeled, minced
- ½ teaspoon xanthan gum

Directions:

1. Add eggs and arrowroot powder into a bowl and whisk well.
2. Add chicken and stir until well coated.
3. Place a large pan over medium flame. Add oil and let it heat. Drop the chicken pieces into the pan, one at a time so that they do not stick together.
4. Cook until golden brown all over.

5. In the meantime, make the sauce mixture by adding coconut aminos, sukrin gold, ginger, 2 tablespoons sesame seeds, sesame oil, vinegar, garlic and xanthan gum into a bowl. Whisk until smooth.
6. Pour the sauce mixture into the pan and stir until well coated. Cook for a couple of minutes. Turn off the heat.
7. Transfer into a large serving bowl. Scatter scallions and remaining sesame seeds on top.
8. You can serve it with steamed cauliflower rice or broccoli.

Keto "Honey" Dinner Recipes

Sesame Beef

Preparation time: 20 minutes

Cooking time: 30 minutes

Number of servings: 8

Nutritional values per serving: 1/8 recipe, without serving options

Calories – 447

Fat – 34 g

Total Carbohydrate – 2 g

Net Carbohydrate – 1 g

Fiber – 1 g

Protein – 33 g

Ingredients:

- 2.2 pounds sirloin steak, cut into strips
- 6 tablespoons oil, divided

- ½ teaspoon black pepper
- 4 cloves garlic, minced
- 2 tablespoons liquid stevia
- 4 tablespoons soy sauce
- 6 spring onions, thinly sliced
- 2 tablespoons sesame seeds

Directions:

1. Combine black pepper, garlic, stevia, soy sauce and sesame seeds in a bowl.
2. Place steak strips and stir until the strips are well coated with the mixture.
3. Cover and set aside for 15 minutes.
4. Place a skillet over high flame. Add half the oil and let the oil heat.
5. Add steak along with the marinade and cook until it is cooked as per your preference.
6. Serve over cauliflower rice or miracle noodles or zucchini noodles.

Keto Beef and Broccoli

Preparation time: 15 minutes

Cooking time: 15 minutes

Number of servings: 2

Nutritional values per serving: ½ the recipe without serving options

Calories – 373

Fat – 20 g

Total Carbohydrate – 8 g

Net Carbohydrate – 6 g

Fiber – 2 g

Protein – 38 g

Ingredients:

For sauce:

- 3 tablespoons low-sodium soy sauce
- ¼ teaspoon Konjac flour or arrowroot flour
- ½ tablespoon keto honey

- ¼ teaspoon red pepper flakes

For stir-fry:

- 5 ounces small broccoli florets
- ½ small onion, sliced
- ½ tablespoon minced ginger root
- ½ tablespoon minced garlic
- 1 tablespoon avocado oil
- ½ pound sirloin strips

To garnish:

- ½ teaspoon sesame seeds
- ½ tablespoon sesame oil

Directions:

1. To make sauce mixture: Add soy sauce, Konjac flour, sweetener and red pepper flakes into a bowl and whisk well.
2. Place broccoli florets in a microwavable bowl. Drizzle a tablespoon of water over it.

3. Cover the bowl and cook on high for 2 – 3 minutes until crisp as well as tender.
4. Drain the broccoli in a colander.
5. Place a skillet over medium-high flame. Add oil and let it heat. Add onion and cook until pink.
6. Stir in ginger and garlic and cook for about half a minute or until you get a nice aroma.
7. Now add the sirloin strips and sauté for not more than 2 minutes. They should have a tinge of pink.
8. Stir the sauce mixture and pour into the skillet. Lower the heat and simmer until thick.
9. Remove the pan from heat and add broccoli. Transfer into a serving dish.
10. Scatter sesame seeds on top. Trickle sesame oil on top and serve.
11. Serve over cauliflower rice or miracle noodles or zucchini noodles.

"Honey" Garlic Meatballs

Preparation time: 10 minutes

Cooking time: 20 minutes

Number of servings: 2

Nutritional values per serving: 4 meatballs with sauce and without pasta

Calories – 649.6

Fat – 43.5 g

Total Carbohydrate – 10.9 g

Net Carbohydrate – 8.2 g

Fiber – 2.7 g

Protein – 51.9 g

Ingredients:

- 1.1 pounds ground beef
- 1 egg
- ¼ teaspoon black pepper

- ½ tablespoon crushed garlic
- ½ tablespoon butter
- ½ tablespoon coconut flour
- ¾ teaspoon salt

For sugar-free ketchup:

- ½ can (from a 6 ounces can) tomato paste
- ½ tablespoon lemon juice
- ¼ teaspoon onion salt
- A pinch black pepper
- ¼ cup water
- 3 – 6 drops stevia or liquid sucralose
- 1/8 teaspoon garlic powder
- 3 tablespoons sugar-free honey
- ½ tablespoon soy sauce (optional)

Directions:

1. You need to prepare the oven and baking sheet: Place rack in the center of the oven. Also make sure that the oven is preheated to 375°F.
2. Take a baking sheet and line it with aluminum foil. Grease the foil sheet with some cooking spray.

3. Add beef and coconut flour into a bowl and mix well.
4. Add egg, pepper and salt into another bowl and whisk well. Pour into the bowl of beef and mix well.
5. Divide the mixture into 8 equal portions and shape into meatballs. Place the meatballs on the baking sheet.
6. Place the baking dish in the oven and bake for 17 – 20 minutes.
7. While the meatballs are baking, make the sugar-free ketchup: Add tomato paste, lemon juice, garlic powder, onion salt, black pepper, water and liquid sweetener into a bowl and whisk well.
8. Whisk in the soy sauce and sugar-free honey.
9. Place a pan over medium flame. Add butter. When butter melts, add garlic and cook for about a minute or until you get a nice aroma.
10. Add meatballs and stir. Pour sauce over the meatballs and mix well. Heat thoroughly.
11. Serve with some keto friendly pasta if desired.

Keto Honey Mustard Salmon

Preparation time: 15 minutes

Cooking time: 50 minutes

Number of servings: 2

Nutritional values per serving:

Salmon with honey mustard sauce | Roasted radishes

(Without broccoli)

Calories – 375 | 91

Fat – 25 g | 8 g

Total Carbohydrate – 0.3 g | 1 g

Net Carbohydrate – 0.3 g | 0.5 g

Fiber – 0 g | 0.5 g

Protein – 34 g | 2

Ingredients:

For keto honey mustard sauce:

- 2 tablespoons Dijon mustard

- 1 tablespoon white wine vinegar
- 2 small cloves garlic, pressed (optional)
- 2 tablespoons allulose or 1 ½ tablespoons erythritol or xylitol
- 2 tablespoons avocado oil
- ½ tablespoon chopped fresh dill (optional)

For salmon:

- 2 salmon fillets
- ½ head broccoli (optional), cut into florets

For roasted radishes:

- 3.5 ounces small to medium radishes, trimmed, halved
- 1 teaspoon minced thyme or ½ teaspoon dried thyme
- Freshly ground pepper to taste
- 1 tablespoon extra-virgin olive oil
- Flaky sea salt to taste
- 2 tablespoons freshly grated parmesan cheese

Directions:

1. To roast radishes: You need to prepare the oven and baking dish: Place rack in the center of the oven. Also make sure that the oven is preheated to 400°F.
2. Take a baking dish and grease it with some cooking spray.
3. Place radishes in the baking dish. Sprinkle thyme, salt and pepper over it. Trickle oil over it. Toss well and spread it evenly.
4. Place the baking dish in the oven and lightly roast the radishes. It should take around 30 minutes. Stir the radishes half way through baking.
5. Scatter Parmesan on top and bake for another 5 minutes.
6. While the radishes are being roasted, make the honey mustard sauce by adding mustard, vinegar and sweetener in a bowl. Whisk well.
7. Pour oil in a thin drizzle, (starting with a couple of drops and then in a thin drizzle) whisking simultaneously. Keep whisking until emulsified. Use an electric hand mixer for whisking.
8. Add dill and garlic and stir. Cover and chill until use. It can last for 4 to 5 days.

9. Meanwhile, prepare a baking sheet by lining it with parchment paper.
10. Increase the temperature of the oven to 450°F.
11. Place fish fillets on the baking sheet, with the skin side facing down.
12. Brush the sauce mixture over the salmon fillets. Be generous with the sauce. Place broccoli florets along with the fish fillets. Spray some cooking spray over the salmon and broccoli. Sprinkle salt and pepper over it.
13. Place the baking dish in the oven and bake for 10 minutes or until the fish flakes easily when pierced with a fork.
14. Serve salmon with broccoli and roasted radishes and of course the remaining sauce mixture.

Keto Honey Garlic Shrimp

Preparation time: 20 minutes

Cooking time: 5 minutes

Number of servings: 2

Nutritional values per serving:

Calories – 599

Fat – 28 g

Total Carbohydrate – 5 g

Net Carbohydrate – 3 g

Fiber – 2 g

Protein – 76 g

Ingredients:

- 1 ½ pounds shrimp, tail on, peeled
- ¼ cup water
- 4 tablespoons soy sauce
- 1 inch fresh ginger, peeled, sliced
- 2 stalks green onion, finely chopped

- 2 tablespoons sesame oil, to fry
- 2 teaspoons sesame oil
- 2 tablespoons swerve or monk fruit sweetener
- 1/8 teaspoon xanthan gum (optional)
- 4 cloves garlic, peeled
- 2 tablespoons chopped almonds (optional)
- 1/8 teaspoon togarashi
- 2 cups cauliflower rice, to serve

Directions:

1. Add garlic and ginger into the small blender jar. Add about a tablespoon of water and blend until smooth.
2. Combine soy sauce, ginger garlic paste, 2 teaspoons sesame oil and togarashi in a large bowl.
3. To make honey mixture: Add sweetener, xanthan gum and water into a small nonstick pan. Place the pan over medium flame. Stir occasionally.
4. When the mixture comes to a boil, lower the heat and cook for a minute. Turn off the heat and transfer into a large bowl.
5. Drop the shrimp into the bowl and stir until shrimp is well coated with the honey mixture. Cover and set aside for 15 minutes.

6. Cook cauliflower rice following the directions on the package.
7. Place a large, nonstick pan over medium flame. Add 2 tablespoons sesame oil and let it heat. Pour the shrimp along with the marinade into the pan. Mix well and spread it evenly on the bottom of the pan.
8. Cover the pan for about 2 to 3 minutes. Uncover and cook until shrimp turns pink.
9. Add green onions and mix well.
10. To serve: Divide cauliflower rice into 2 plates. Divide shrimp among the plates.
11. Scatter togarashi and almonds on top and serve.

Keto Honey Glazed Salmon

Preparation time: 10 minutes

Cooking time: 15 minutes

Number of servings: 2

Nutritional values per serving:

Calories – 253

Fat –17.4 g

Total Carbohydrate – 5.1 g

Net Carbohydrate – 3.7 g

Fiber – 1.4 g

Protein – 38.4 g

Ingredients:

- ½ tablespoon avocado oil
- ½ teaspoon salt
- 2 skin-on center-cut salmon fillets (6 ounces each)

For sauce:

- ½ tablespoon avocado oil
- ½ tablespoon Dijon mustard
- ½ teaspoon grated, fresh ginger
- ¼ teaspoon red pepper flakes
- Zest of ½ lime, grated
- 1 tablespoon tamari
- 1 tablespoon brown erythritol or swerve
- 2 small cloves garlic, peeled, minced
- ¼ teaspoon white pepper
- Juice of ½ lime

For garnish:

- ½ tablespoon chopped cilantro
- Few lime slices
- 1 tablespoon thinly sliced green onion

Directions:

1. Place a skillet over medium-high flame. Add oil and let it heat.
2. Sprinkle salt over the salmon and lay it down in the skillet, with the skin touching the bottom of the skillet.

3. Do not disturb the salmon for about 5 to 6 minutes. By now the skin should not be sticking to the pan. Turn the salmon over and cook for 5 to 6 minutes or until salmon is cooked through. Remove salmon from the pan and set it aside on a plate.
4. Add oil, mustard, ginger, red pepper flakes, lemon zest, tamari, brown erythritol, garlic, white pepper and lime juice into the skillet. Whisk well and constantly until thick.
5. Add salmon into the skillet. Take a spoon and pour the sauce over salmon.
6. Sprinkle cilantro and green onion on top. Place a few lime slices on top and serve.

Keto Honey Garlic Chicken with Charred Peppers

Preparation time: 20 minutes

Cooking time: 20 minutes

Number of servings: 3

Nutritional values per serving: Without serving options

Calories – 585

Fat – 58 g

Total Carbohydrate – 15 g

Net Carbohydrate – 6.7 g

Fiber – 3 g

Protein – 72 g

Ingredients:

- 1 ½ pounds chicken breasts, thaw if frozen, cut into pieces
- 1/3 allulose
- ¼ teaspoon cayenne pepper
- 1 tablespoon coconut aminos
- Avocado oil or olive oil

- 1 ½ bell peppers, deseeded, sliced
- ¼ cup water
- Black pepper to taste
- 2 tablespoons rice vinegar
- Salt to taste

Serving options:

- Cauliflower rice
- Steamed broccoli

Directions:

1. Combine allulose, rice vinegar, salt, water, coconut aminos and cayenne pepper into a saucepan and whisk well.
2. Place the saucepan over medium flame. Stir often and let the mixture come to a rolling boil.
3. Lower the heat and simmer until slightly thick. Turn off the heat.
4. Place a skillet over medium-high flame. Add a little oil (about a tablespoon) and let it heat.
5. Add bell peppers and cook until bell peppers are brownish- blackish. Transfer the peppers into a bowl.
6. Season chicken with salt and pepper and add into the skillet along with a tablespoon of oil.

7. Sear the chicken until golden brown all over. Lower the heat to medium-low.
8. Pour the keto honey – garlic sauce mixture into the pan of chicken and mix well.
9. Serve keto honey garlic chicken with charred peppers and serving options if desired.

Asian "Honey" Chicken

Preparation time: 10 minutes

Cooking time: 20 minutes

Number of servings: 6

Nutritional values per serving: 1/3 cup, without serving options

Calories – 220

Fat – 10 g

Total Carbohydrate – 2 g

Net Carbohydrate – 2 g

Fiber – 0 g

Protein – 22 g

Ingredients:

For the chicken:

- 2 pounds chicken breasts, chopped into chunks
- Freshly ground black pepper to taste
- 1/8 teaspoon Himalayan pink salt or to taste

For the sauce:

- ½ cup water
- 2/3 cup Lakanato golden monk fruit sweetener
- 2 teaspoons crushed red pepper
- 6 tablespoons liquid aminos
- 2 teaspoons sesame oil
- 1 teaspoon xanthan gum

Serving options:

- Cooked cauliflower rice
- Zucchini noodles

Directions:

1. Sprinkle salt and pepper over the chicken.
2. Place a large nonstick pan over medium-high flame. Add chicken into the pan and stir occasionally until chicken is well cooked inside. Transfer into a bowl.
3. To make sauce: Add water, sweetener, crushed pepper, liquid aminos and sesame oil into the pan and stir. When the mixture begins to boil, sprinkle xanthan gum on top and whisk well.

4. Add the chicken back into the pan and simmer until the sauce is thickened to suit your taste.
5. Serve with cauliflower rice or zucchini noodles if desired.

Keto Sweet and Sour Chicken

Preparation time: 25 minutes

Cooking time: 25 minutes

Number of servings: 3

Nutritional values per serving:

Calories – 458

Fat – 29.6 g

Total Carbohydrate – 11.4 g

Net Carbohydrate – 7.6 g

Fiber – 3.8 g

Protein – 36 g

Ingredients:

For the chicken:

- ¾ pound chicken breast or chicken thighs, cut into 2 inch cubes
- 1 egg
- 1/8 teaspoon salt or to taste

- 1 tablespoon plain, unsweetened almond milk or coconut milk
- 1 ounce whey protein isolate
- 1 ½ cups avocado oil or algae oil, to fry

For the stir-fry:

- ½ green bell pepper, cut into 1 inch square pieces
- ½ red bell pepper, cut into 1 inch square pieces
- 1 medium yellow onion, cut into 1 inch square pieces

For sauce mixture:

- ¼ cup granulated erythritol
- ¼ cup distilled vinegar
- ½ tablespoon tamari
- 2 tablespoons brown erythritol
- 3 tablespoons unsweetened ketchup or any sugar-free ketchup
- 1 clove garlic, peeled, minced

To serve:

- 1 green onion, thinly sliced
- 3 cups cauliflower rice

Directions:

1. Crack egg into a bowl. Add milk and whisk well.
2. Place whey protein isolate and salt in another bowl and stir well.
3. Place a deep fryer pan over medium flame. Add oil. The oil should cover at least 2 inches in height from the bottom of the pan so add more oil if required. Let the oil heat to 350° F.
4. While the oil is heating, dunk the chicken pieces in the egg mixture, one at a time.
5. Remove the chicken piece and shake off excess egg. Dredge the chicken piece in whey protein isolate mixture and add into the hot oil. Add only as many that can fit in the pan. Do not overcrowd.
6. Cook until golden brown. Remove chicken with a slotted spoon and place on a plate lined with layers of paper towels.
7. Cook the remaining chicken in batches similarly.
8. Retain a tablespoon of oil in the pan and remove the remaining oil.
9. Add onion and bell pepper into the pan and cook until slightly tender.

10. Add granulated erythritol, vinegar, tamari, brown erythritol, ketchup and garlic and stir until well combined.
11. Stir often until the sauce is slightly thick.
12. Add chicken into the pan and heat thoroughly.
13. Serve with steamed cauliflower rice, garnished with green onions.

Keto "Honey" Dessert Recipes

Keto Holiday "Honey" Cake

Preparation time: 15 minutes

Cooking time: 25 – 30 minutes

Number of servings: 8

Nutritional values per serving:

Calories – 165

Fat – 7 g

Total Carbohydrate – 3 g

Net Carbohydrate – 1 g

Fiber – 2 g

Protein – 5 g

Ingredients:

- 1 1/3 cups superfine almond flour
- ¼ teaspoon Himalayan pink salt
- 1/8 teaspoon ground allspice

- ½ teaspoon baking soda
- ½ tablespoon ground cinnamon
- 1/8 teaspoon ground cloves
- ¼ cup lakanato sweetener
- ½ tablespoons freshly brewed liquid espresso
- ¼ cup coconut oil
- 2 eggs
- 1 tablespoon slivered almonds

Directions:

1. You need to prepare the oven and loaf pan: Place rack in the center of the oven. Also make sure that the oven is preheated to 350°F.
2. Grease a small loaf pan with some cooking spray.
3. To mix the dry ingredients: Add almond flour, salt, allspice, baking soda, cinnamon and cloves into a mixing bowl and stir well.
4. Add sweetener, liquid espresso, coconut oil and eggs and whisk until you get a smooth batter.
5. Pour the batter into the prepared loaf pan. Scatter almonds on top.

6. Place the loaf pan in the oven and bake for 25 – 30 minutes or until a toothpick when inserted in the center of the cake comes out without any particles stuck on it.
7. Cut into 8 equal slices and serve.

Keto Pumpkin Coffee Cake with Honey Butter

Preparation time: 15 minutes

Cooking time: 40 – 50 minutes

Number of servings: 18

Nutritional values per serving:

Calories – 570

Fat – 53 g

Total Carbohydrate – 9 g

Net Carbohydrate – 3 g

Fiber – 6 g

Protein – 11 g

Ingredients:

For the cake:

- 4 egg yolks
- 2 eggs
- 1 cup heavy cream, chilled
- 1 teaspoon vanilla extract

- 4 teaspoons pumpkin pie spice
- ½ cup lakanto powdered monk fruit sweetener
- 2 teaspoons liquid stevia
- ½ cup coconut flour
- 2 cups almond flour
- 1 cup pumpkin puree
- 1/8 teaspoon salt
- 2 teaspoons baking powder

For crumble:

- 4 cups almond flour
- 4 teaspoons pumpkin pie spice
- 1 cup butter, melted
- ½ cup lakanto granulated monk fruit sweetener
- 1 teaspoon sea salt
- 1 cup chopped pecans

For honey butter:

- ½ cup lakanto powdered monk fruit sweetener
- 1 cup butter, at room temperature
- 1 teaspoon liquid stevia

Directions:

1. To make cake: You need to prepare the oven and baking pan: Place rack in the center of the oven. Also make sure that the oven is preheated to 350°F.
2. Grease a baking pan with some cooking spray.
3. Add heavy cream and sweetener into a mixing bowl and whisk with an electric hand mixer until stiff peaks are just formed.
4. Add eggs, yolks, vanilla, pumpkin pie spice, salt, baking powder, almond flour, coconut flour, stevia and pumpkin puree and whisk until just combined. Few lumps may be visible, but that is OK. Scrape the sides of the bowl whenever required.
5. Pour the batter into the baking pan.
6. To make crumble: Add almond flour, pumpkin pie spice, butter, sweetener, salt and pecans in a bowl and mix until crumbly in texture.
7. Scatter the crumble mixture on top of the batter.
8. Place the baking pan in the oven and bake for 40 – 45 minutes or until a toothpick when inserted in the center of the cake, has no particles stuck on in when removed.
9. The top should be slightly brown.

10. To make honey butter: While the cake is baking, add butter, stevia and monk fruit sweetener into a bowl and mix well.
11. When the cake is done, remove the baking pan from the oven and let it cool until warm.
12. Cut into 18 equal slices and serve topped with honey butter.

Keto Vanilla Pudding with "Honey"

Preparation time: 5 minutes

Cooking time: 5 minutes

Number of servings: 8

Nutritional values per serving:

Calories – 260

Fat – 21 g

Total Carbohydrate – 5.4 g

Net Carbohydrate – 3.2 g

Fiber – 2.2 g

Protein – 6.4 g

Ingredients:

- 3 cups sour cream
- 2 tablespoons vanilla extract
- 4 tablespoons dark cocoa powder
- 8 micro scoops 100% stevia extract
- 2/3 cup keto honey

To top:

- 1 teaspoon ground cinnamon
- 8 pieces walnuts

Directions:

1. Add sour cream and keto honey into a saucepan. Place the saucepan over medium flame. Whisk until well incorporated.
2. Stir in the vanilla and cook for about 4 minutes. Stirring frequently. Turn off the heat.
3. Immerse a cup in hot water for a couple of minutes and remove it.
4. Add about ½ cup of the sour cream mixture into the hot cup. Add cocoa into the cup and whisk until smooth.
5. Spoon remaining sour cream mixture into 8 decorative glasses.
6. Divide the cocoa mixture among the glasses.
7. Sprinkle cinnamon on top. Place a piece of walnut in each glass and refrigerate for 3 – 6 hours.
8. Serve chilled.

Baklava Cookies

Preparation time: 15 minutes

Cooking time: 35 minutes

Number of servings: 12

Nutritional values per serving: 1 cookie

Calories – 109

Fat – 10 g

Total Carbohydrate – 3 g

Net Carbohydrate – 2 g

Fiber – 1 g

Protein – 1 g

Ingredients:

For pastry dough:

- 1.5 ounces cream cheese, softened
- 3 tablespoons coconut flour
- 3 tablespoons almond flour
- 2 ounces butter, softened

- Yolk of a small egg
- 3 tablespoons ground golden flaxseeds

For the filling:

- ¼ teaspoon ground cinnamon
- 6 tablespoons chopped nuts of your choice

For syrup:

- ¼ cup Trim Healthy Mama Gentle Sweet
- 2 strips lemon zest (1 inch each)
- ½ tablespoon water
- 1 ½ tablespoons keto honey

Directions:

1. You need to prepare the oven and mini muffin pan: Place rack in the center of the oven. Also make sure that the oven is preheated to 350°F.
2. Grease a mini muffin pan with some cooking spray.
3. To make dough: Add cream cheese, coconut flour, almond flour, butter, yolk and flaxseeds into a bowl and mix until dough is formed.

4. Make 12 equal portions of the dough and place them in the wells of the muffin pan. Press them onto the bottom of the pan.
5. To make nut filling: Add cinnamon and nuts into a bowl and stir. Divide the nut mixture equally and sprinkle over the dough, in the mini muffin pan.
6. Place the mini muffin pan in an oven and bake until the cookies are golden brown. It should take around 20 to 23 minutes anyway keep a watch on the cookies after 15 minutes of baking.
7. While the cookies are baking, the syrup can be prepared. For this, add water, cinnamon, sweetener and lemon zest strips into a small saucepan.
8. Place the saucepan over medium-low flame. When the mixture begins to boil, lower the heat and cook for 2 – 3 minutes or until slightly thick, like syrup.
9. Turn off the heat and let it cool. Add keto honey and stir. Trickle this mixture over the cookies in the muffin pan. Let it rest for a few minutes.
10. Take out the cookies from the muffin pan and serve.

Keto Baklava

Preparation time: 15 minutes

Cooking time: 40 – 50 minutes

Number of servings: 10

Nutritional values per serving:

Calories – 150

Fat – 13 g

Total Carbohydrate – 5.7 g

Net Carbohydrate – 1.7 g

Fiber – 4 g

Protein – 3.8 g

Ingredients:

For dough:

- 3 large egg whites
- 1.5 ounces chia seeds
- 2 ½ tablespoons powdered erythritol
- ½ tablespoon psyllium husks

For the filling:

- 2.5 ounces walnuts, finely chopped
- 3 large egg yolks
- 2 ounces butter, melted
- ¼ teaspoon ground cinnamon
- 1 ounce full-fat coconut milk
- 1 tablespoon powdered erythritol

For the syrup:

- 3 tablespoons water
- ½ tablespoon grated orange zest
- 2 tablespoons keto honey
- 3 tablespoons erythritol
- 5 drops orange oil (optional)

Directions:

1. You need to prepare the oven and baking sheet: Place rack in the center of the oven. Also make sure that the oven is preheated to 390°F.
2. Place a sheet of parchment paper on a baking sheet.
3. To make dough: Add egg whites into a mixing bowl. Beat with an electric hand mixer until nice and frothy.

4. Beat in the erythritol. Keep beating until stiff peaks are formed.
5. Add chia seeds and psyllium husks and stir lightly with a spatula.
6. Spread the batter on the baking sheet. Place the baking sheet in the oven and set the timer for 10 minutes.
7. Once baked, remove the baking sheet from the oven and let it cool completely.
8. Peel off the parchment paper. Cut the dough into 3 equal parts (rectangular in shape).
9. Take a baking dish that can fit a dough rectangle in it. Spread some melted butter in the baking dish, on the bottom as well as the sides.
10. Adjust the temperature of the oven to 325°F.
11. To fill and layer: Place one dough rectangle in the baking dish.
12. Add cinnamon and walnuts in a small bowl and stir.
13. Add yolks into another bowl and whisk well. Add melted butter, coconut milk and a tablespoon of erythritol.
14. Spread 1/3 of the yolk mixture over the dough in the baking dish. Sprinkle half the walnuts and cinnamon.
15. Place one more dough rectangle over it.

16. Repeat steps 14 – 15 once again. Spread remaining yolk mixture on the top dough rectangle.
17. Cut the baklava into the shapes of parallelograms. You should have 10 equal sized parallelograms.
18. Place the baking dish in the oven and set the timer for 30 minutes or until light golden brown on top.
19. To make syrup: Add water, orange zest, keto honey and erythritol into a saucepan.
20. Place the saucepan over medium flame. When it begins to boil, lower the flame and simmer until slightly thick. Turn off the heat. Add orange oil if using and stir.
21. Remove the baked baklava from the oven and drizzle hot syrup over the baklava right away.
22. Cool completely, without covering.
23. Serve.

Conclusion

Thank you for purchasing the book.

Most people wonder if honey can be consumed on a keto diet. While it is true that honey has carbs, it has numerous health benefits. Honey is rich in minerals and nutrients and is quite easy for the body to digest. Honey is a substitute for sugar, and though it contains the same sugar molecules as sugar, it is easier for the body to digest it because of the enzyme present. This means our body does not store the sugar molecules but burns them to produce energy.

If you enjoy sweet food, you will love the recipes in the book. They do not use sugar, but honey, and the food tastes the same, maybe even better. The instructions are easy to follow, and you have the nutrition value against each recipe. So, choose the dish depending on the number of calories you want to eat.

I hope you and your family enjoy the recipes in the book.

www.ingramcontent.com/pod-product-compliance
Lightning Source LLC
Chambersburg PA
CBHW071526080526
44588CB00011B/1571